The Pescatarian Cookbook

The Complete Pescatarian Cookbook with 50 Flavorful and Simple Fish Recipes to Help You Maintain a Healthy Lifestyle

The Inspirational Chef

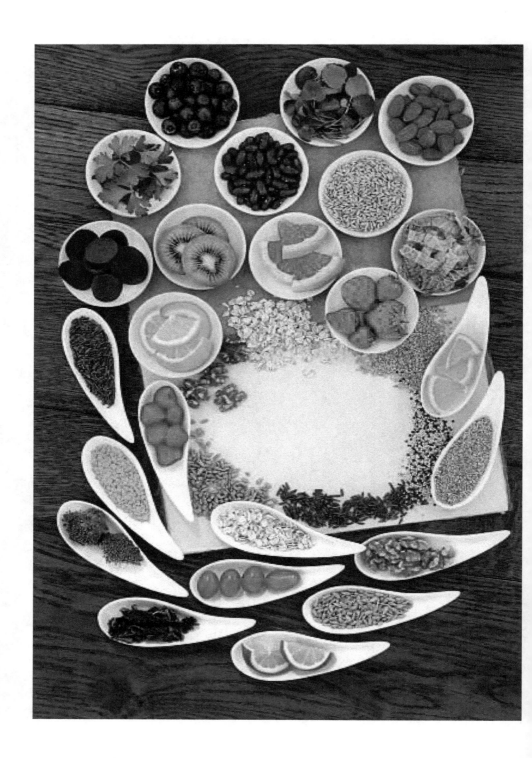

Table of Content

Introduction

In recent times, a lot of attention has been drawn to sustainability and preserving the earth. Global population growth and increased life expectancy mean there are growing concerns about how to feed the world's population. In response to this, growth boosters are being used for animal production and preservatives used to maintain plant foods. This has led to an increase in heart disease, diabetes, and cancer. This new reality has caused a lot of the world's population to seek ways to eat healthy while preserving the planet. For some, it is switching to veganism, for others it is pescatarianism.

The word 'pescatarian' was created in the early 1990s. It is a combination of the Italian word for fish – *pesce* – and vegetarian. A pescatarian is anyone who eats a plant-based diet, along with fish and seafood. A pescatarian may also eat dairy products and eggs. They do not, however, eat any form of animal meat. A pescatarian still gets the bulk of his or her food from plant sources such as whole grains, legumes, nuts, fruits, and vegetables. They are usually people who want all the great benefits of a plant-based diet, as well as the healthy nutrients from fish.

You might be wondering whether eating fish and seafood negates the aim of vegetarianism. The answer is, not entirely. Pescatarians usually forgo meat in their diet for environmental and ethical reasons, just as a vegetarian would.
And they get similar results too. A pescatarian diet is helpful for weight loss and a healthy lifestyle, as studies have shown.

Fish contains omega-3 fatty acid, high-quality protein, and low fat. It is a much better source of protein than meat. A fish diet such as the Mediterranean diet or the Atkins diet has been linked to a reduced rate of heart disease, stroke and ultimately death from these diseases. Fish is also rich in vitamin B2 (riboflavin), and vitamin D, provides minerals like phosphorus and calcium, and offers variety in taste and recipes! In addition, it is essential for pregnant women as it aids the development of fetal vision and the nervous system. Its benefits for adults also include brain health.

But it is not all Kumbaya when it comes to eating fish and seafood as they can be contaminated. Some fish high in mercury include shark, tilefish, and swordfish, and these should be avoided. Larger fish tend to have more mercury than smaller ones.

In this book, we have avoided all fish that tend to contain mercury and are going to discuss ways to make fish into delicious meals. But first, let us look in more detail at some of the reasons people opt for pescatarianism:

Health factors

A plant-based diet with fish and seafood included offers a large variety of nutrients and options. Save for some legumes and nuts, a plant-based diet has more carbs than protein and getting one's protein requirement means consuming a large portion of these protein plants.

This can be quite exhausting. But with a pescatarian diet, you get healthy nutrients from grains, fruits, and legumes as well as lean protein from fish.

Environmental factors

According to a report by the UN, raising livestock increases the earth's carbon emissions by as much as 15%. Seafood, on the other hand, has a much lower carbon footprint than livestock. Studies carried out in 2014 have shown that people who eat seafood create 46% less greenhouse gas emissions than meat eaters. It also showed that producing cheese and animal meat has a higher carbon footprint than the production of seafood.

Ethical reasons

A lot of people who think of going vegan for ethical reasons but do not think they can get all their protein from plant sources settle for pescatarianism. Some of these ethical reasons could be the inhumane and crude way some slaughterhouses kill the animals, or generally being against the killing of animals.

Sometimes they are opposed to the conditions under which these animals are raised.

Another ethical reason could be the poor working conditions of slaughterhouse workers. Some pescatarians also believe it is a waste of land and resources to raise grains for the feeding of livestock when there is so much hunger in the world.

Are fish not caught under the same inhumane conditions you may ask? The answer is, not really. The aquaculture and fishing industries have taken steps to ensure fish are raised and caught in the most humane way possible. In Alaska, for example, fishing companies ensure there is no disruption in the fish population by ensuring only adult males are caught.

Benefits of a pescatarian diet

The benefits of a pescatarian diet are immense. It is a combination of the benefits of a plant-based diet and seafood, a balanced diet plan. A pescatarian diet answers the concerns some people might have about getting the required nutrients from just plant sources. Seafood is rich in B vitamins, especially vitamins B12, zinc, calcium and protein, nutrients that are hard to get from a plant-based diet.

Omega-3 fatty acid

Fish is famous for its omega-3 fatty acid. Although some plant food sources such as walnut and flaxseed contain a type of omega-3 fat, alpha-linolenic acid (ALA), it is not easily convertible by the body into eicosapentaenoic acid (EPA) and docosahexaenoic acid (DHA) which are great for the heart, the brain and one's mood. Fish such as salmon and sardines on the other hand contain both EPA and DHA.

Boost's protein intake

Getting lean protein from plant sources is not so easy as it usually comes with carbs, and to get the required amount of protein, one must eat a large portion of food. As humans, we need about 0.8 grams of protein for every kilogram of our body weight. That means a person who is 50kg will need 40 grams of protein daily. Some people like to eat more protein than the required amount. Getting this protein from plant sources is hard, especially if you do not want extra carbs.

Thankfully, fish and other seafood are packed with lean protein. Whitefish such as cod, halibut, flounder, or haddock contain 18 grams of protein in every ounce (28). Shrimp on the other hand delivers 12 grams of protein in every 3 ounces while tuna delivers 25 grams of protein in the same. Tilapia, a popular and inexpensive fish, contains 23 grams of protein in every 3 ounces.

The great part about fish is that they are very filling, so you do not need to eat a lot to get satisfied.

Access to more nutrients

It is not just lean protein you get from a fish diet. You also get a lot of other nutrients. Some seafood such as oysters are very high in vitamin B12, selenium and zinc. This is so high that one oyster gives about 130% of the RDI for vitamin B12 and 55% of the RDI for zinc and selenium. Shrimps are rich in choline, niacin, zinc, selenium, and vitamins E, B6 and B12.

They are also high in astaxanthin, an antioxidant that reduces oxidative and inflammatory damage. Mussels contain high quantities of vitamin B12 and the other B vitamins as well as selenium and manganese.

Access to more food options

Every vegetarian knows the diet can be quite limiting, and eating in regular restaurants can be a hassle, as the best you can get in most cases is cheesy pasta. But with a pescatarian diet, you will have access to oysters, shrimp and fish which can be grilled, sautéed, and baked.

Reduces the chance of heart disease

Fish and seafood contain omega-3 fatty acid which is great for the heart. There is strong evidence that eating fish and taking fish oil is good for the heart. They are so good that they get a nod from the American Heart Association, which recommends eating fish at least twice a week. How does fish work for the heart? Fish contains omega-3 fatty acid which reduces inflammation in the body. This also includes inflammation that can damage the blood vessels and lead to stroke and other heart diseases.

Omega-3 fatty acids benefit the heart by decreasing triglycerides, slightly lowering blood pressure, reducing irregular heartbeats, and reducing blood clotting.

Fish high in omega-3 fatty acids include Atlantic mackerel, cod, herring, lake trout, salmon, sardines, and tuna. However, tuna contains some amount of mercury. Although this is countered by its high selenium content, tuna should be eaten in moderation.

How to shop and store seafood

Now that we have established that seafood is great for you, how do you shop for and store it? Fish, unlike plant foods, is highly perishable and improper storage can taint its taste. The first thing to know is that fish and seafood have a short shelf life so you will have to shop for them quite frequently.

Here are a few things to take into consideration when buying fish and seafood:

When shopping for fish and seafood in a supermarket, look out for the Marine Stewardship Council (MSC) sticker.

The sticker indicates that the fish has come from sustainable fisheries and your purchase will be helping the environment.

Eat a variety of fish. There is already a large demand for certain fish species such as Atlantic cod and salmon, and these are therefore overfished. Going with other fish varieties will be helpful to both your pocket and the environment. Anchovies, abalone clams, crayfish, hake, farmed mussels and oysters are all tasty sustainable choices.

Buy local. If possible, buy fish caught by your local fisheries. This means they are fresh and have not travelled from halfway across the world to your supermarket.

When shopping, buy your fish and seafood just before you leave the supermarket. This way they do not stay out of the fridge or freezer for too long.

Keep your fish and seafood bloodless and in the coldest part of your freezer or refrigerator. Jot down the date each was kept in the freezer, so it does not stay in there too long and lose its taste. It is not ideal to freeze fish for more than 3 months, and prawns and shrimps for more than 6 months. Also take into consideration the time it spent in the supermarket before your purchase.

Now that you are well caught up on the fundamentals of the pescatarian diet, let us dig in to some healthy and yummy recipes.

10-day Meal Plan

Day	Breakfast	Lunch	Dinner
Monday	Plum Muffins	Cremini Mushroom Risotto	Simple Pizza Recipe
Tuesday	Omelet	Old Fashion Pilaf	Squash Quiche
Wednesday	Chocolate Chip Banana Pancake	Risotto with Vegetables	Red Onion Frittata
Thursday	Breakfast Burrito	Polenta with Mushrooms and Chickpeas	Tomato and Onion Pasta
Friday	Sweet Potato Skillet	Turmeric Tempeh Stir-Fry	Cheese Frittata
Saturday	Overnight Chocolate Chia Pudding	Cauliflower, Navy Beans and Quinoa Risotto	Couscous Salad
Sunday	Vanilla Buckwheat Porridge	Butternut Squash with Quinoa and Almonds	Cheese Macaroni
Monday	Flaxseed Yogurt	Harissa Lentils with Rice Cauliflower	Broccoli Frittata
Tuesday	Broccoli omelet	Lemony Farro and Pine Nut Chard Rolls	Dried Tomato Salad
Wednesday	Pumpkin French Toast	Rice With Almonds, Parsley And Cranberries	Cauliflower & Farro Salad

Breakfast

Plum Muffins

Preparation Time: 10 Minutes
Cooking Time: 20 Minutes
Total Time: 30 Minutes
Serves: 8-12

Ingredients

- 2 eggs -
- 1 tablespoon olive oil -
- 1 cup milk -
- 2 cups whole wheat flour -
- 1 tsp baking soda -
- ¼ tsp baking soda -
- 1 tsp cinnamon -
- 1 cup plums

Instructions

1. In a bowl combine all wet ingredients
2. In another bowl combine all dry ingredients
3. Combine wet and dry ingredients together
4. Pour mixture into 8-12 prepared muffin cups, fill 2/3 of the cups
5. Bake for 18-20 minutes at 375 F
6. When ready remove from the oven and serve

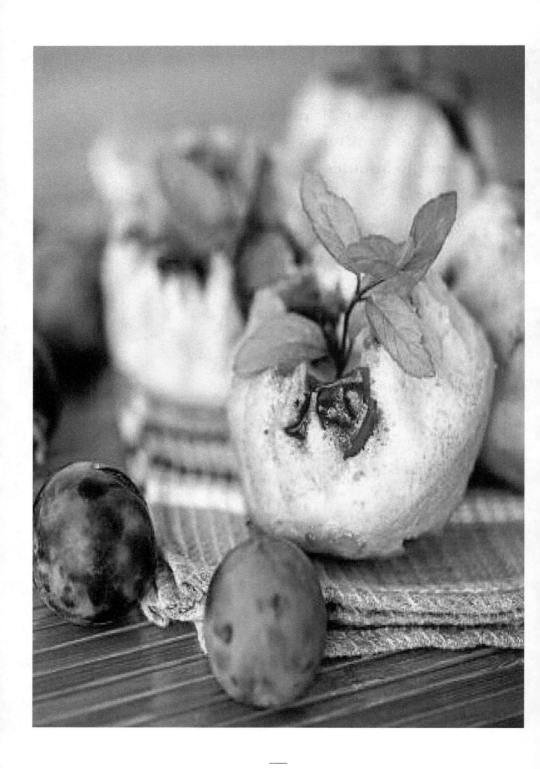

Omelet

Preparation time: 5 minutes

Cooking time: 10 minutes

Total time: 15 minutes

Serves: 1

Ingredients

- 2 eggs -
- ¼ tsp salt -
- ¼ tsp black pepper -
- 1 tablespoon olive oil -
- ¼ cup cheese -
- ¼ tsp basil

Instructions

1. In a bowl combine all ingredients together and mix well
2. In a skillet heat olive oil and pour the egg mixture
3. Cook for 1-2 minutes per side
4. When ready remove omelet from the skillet and serve

Breakfast Burrito

Preparation Time: 5 Minutes
Cooking Time: 15 minutes
Servings: 2

Ingredients

- ½ block (7 ounces) firm tofu
- Two medium potatoes, cut into ¼-inch dice
- 1 cup cooked black beans that should be drained and rinsed
- 4 ounces mushrooms, sliced
- One jalapeño, seeded and diced
- Two tablespoons vegetable broth or water
- One tablespoon nutritional yeast
- ½ teaspoon garlic powder
- ½ teaspoon onion powder
- ¼ cup of salsa
- Six corn tortillas

Instructions

1. Heat a large skillet over medium-low heat.

2. Drain the tofu, then place it in the pan and mash it down with a fork or mixing spoon.

3. Stir the potatoes, black beans, mushrooms, jalapeño, broth, nutritional yeast, garlic powder, and onion powder into the skillet. Change and maintain the heat to low, cover, and cook for 10 minutes, or up wait till the potatoes can be easily punctured with a fork.

4. Uncover, and stir in the salsa. Cook for 5 minutes, stirring every other minute.

5. Thaw the tortillas in a microwave for 15 to 30 seconds or in a warm oven until soft.

6. Remove the pan from the heat. Fill in the center of each tortilla.

7. Roll the tortillas into burritos before serving.

Nutrition Information

Calories: 5.5; Total fat: 8g; Carbohydrates: 95g; Protein: 29g

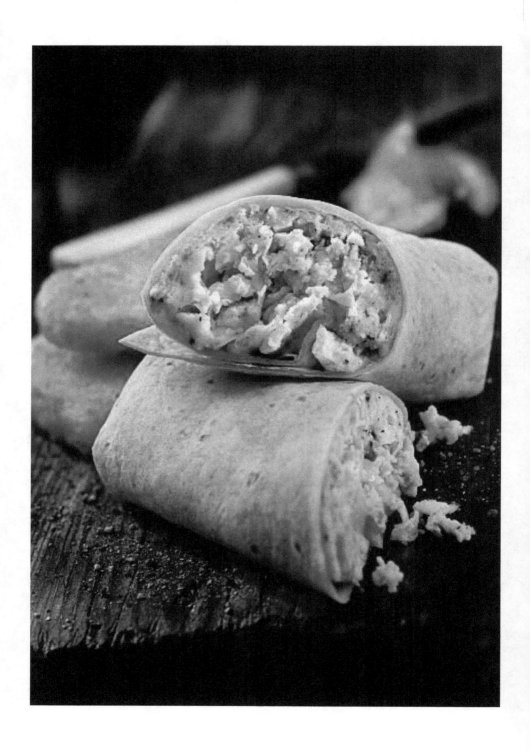

Sweet Potato Skillet

Preparation Time: 5 Minutes
Cooking Time: 15 Minutes
Servings: 4
Ingredients

- Four medium sweet potatoes, cut into ½-inch dice

- 8 ounces' mushrooms, sliced

- One bell pepper, diced

- One sweet onion, diced

- 1 cup vegetable broth or water, then add 1 to 2 tablespoons more if needed

- One teaspoon garlic powder

- ½ teaspoon ground cumin

- ½ teaspoon chili powder

- ⅛ Teaspoon freshly ground black pepper

Instructions

1. Heat a large skillet over medium-low heat.
2. When the skillet is hot, put the sweet potatoes, mushrooms, bell pepper, onion, broth, garlic powder, cumin, chili powder, and pepper in it and stir—cover and cook for 10 minutes.
3. Stir the mixture well. (If any of the contents are beginning to stick to the bottom of the pan, just add 1 to 2 tablespoons of broth.)
4. For an additional 5 minutes, cook it uncovered and stirring once after about 2½ minutes, and serve

Nutrition Information

Calories: 158; Total fat: 1g; Carbohydrates: 34g; Protein: 6g

Vanilla Buckwheat Porridge

Preparation Time: 5 Minutes
Cooking Time: 25 Minutes
Servings: 4

Ingredients

- 3 cups of water
- 1 cup raw buckwheat groats
- One teaspoon ground cinnamon
- One banana, sliced
- ¼ cup golden raisins
- ¼ cup dried currants
- ¼ cup sunflower seeds
- Two tablespoons chia seeds
- One tablespoon hemp seed
- One tablespoon sesame seed, toasted
- ½ cup unsweetened nondairy milk
- One tablespoon pure maple syrup
- One teaspoon vanilla extract

Instructions

1. Boil the water in a pot. Stir in the buckwheat, cinnamon, and banana. Cook the mixture. Mixing it and wait for it to boil, then reduce the heat to medium-low.

2. Cover the pot and cook for 15 minutes, or until the buckwheat is tender. Remove from the heat.

3. Stir in the raisins, currants, sunflower seeds, chia seeds, hemp seeds, sesame seeds, milk, maple syrup, and vanilla. Cover the pot.

4. Wait for 10 minutes before serving.

5. Serve as is or top as desired.

Nutrition Information

Calories: 353; Fats: 11g; Carbohydrates: 61g; Protein: 10g

Flaxseed Yogurt

Preparation Time: 5 Minutes

Cooking Time: 0 Minutes

Servings: 4

Ingredients

- 2 Cups Water
- ½ Cup Hemp Seeds
- 2 Teaspoons Psyllium Husk
- 1 Cup Almond Milk
- ½ Cup Flaxseeds
- ¼ Cup Lemon Juice, Fresh
- ¼ Teaspoon Stevia

Instructions

1. Soak your flaxseed according to package instruction, and then drain the water. Add a cup of boiling water to a blender, and then add in all ingredients. Blend for four minutes.
2. Pour a cup of water in psyllium husk and almond milk. Blend for another half a minute.
3. Add the lemon juice and stevia, blending a little more. Pour in the flaxseed yogurt into containers, and then serve chilled. It will keep for three days in the fridge or sixty in the freezer.

Broccoli omelet

Preparation Time: 5 Minutes
Cooking Time: 10 Minutes
Total Time: 15 Minutes
Serves: 1

Ingredients

- 2 eggs -
- ¼ tsp salt -
- ¼ tsp black pepper -
- 1 tablespoon olive oil -
- ¼ cup cheese -
- ¼ tsp basil -
- 1 cup broccoli

Instructions

1. In a bowl combine all ingredients together and mix well
2. In a skillet heat olive oil and pour the egg mixture
3. Cook for 1-2 minutes per side
4. When ready remove omelet from the skillet and serve

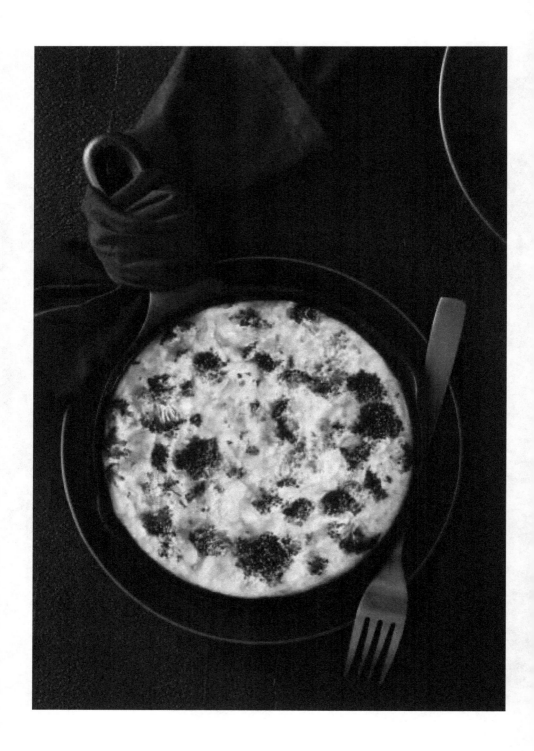

Pumpkin French Toast

Preparation Time: 5 Minutes
Cooking Time: 15 Minutes
Total Time: 20 Minutes
Serves: 3

Ingredients

- ¼ cup milk -
- 2 eggs -
- ½ cup pumpkin puree -
- 1 tablespoon pumpkin slice -
- 6 bread slices

Instructions

1. In a bowl whisk all ingredients for the dipping
2. Dip the bread into the dipping and let it soak for 3-4 minutes
3. In a skillet heat olive oil and fry each slice for 2-3 minutes per side
4. When ready remove from the skillet and serve

Lunch

Cremini Mushroom Risotto

Preparation Time: 5 Minutes
Cooking Time: 15 Minutes
Servings: 3
Ingredients

- 3 tablespoons vegan butter
- 1 teaspoon garlic, minced
- 1 teaspoon thyme
- 1 pound Cremini mushrooms, sliced
- 1 ½ cups white rice
- 2 ½ cups vegetable broth
- 1/4 cup dry sherry wine
- Kosher salt and ground black pepper, to taste
- 3 tablespoons fresh scallions, thinly sliced

Instructions

1. In a saucepan, melt the vegan butter over a moderately high flame. Cook the garlic and thyme for about 1 minute or until aromatic.
2. Add in the mushrooms and continue to sauté until they release the liquid or about 3 minutes.
3. Add in the rice, vegetable broth and sherry wine. Bring to a boil; immediately turn the heat to a gentle simmer.
4. Cook for about 15 minutes or until all the liquid has absorbed. Fluff the rice with a fork, season with salt and pepper and garnish with fresh scallions.
5. Bon appétit!

Nutrition Information

Calories: 513; Protein: 11.7g; Carbohydrates: 88g; Fat: 12.5g

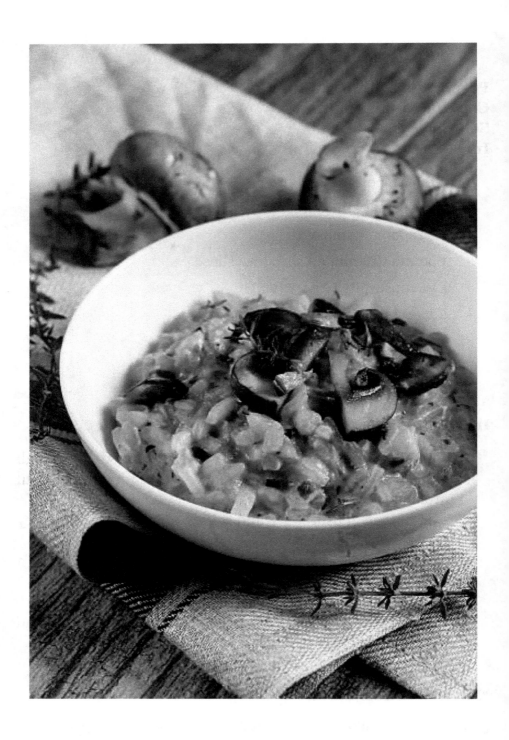

Risotto with Vegetables

Preparation Time: 10 Minutes
Cooking Time: 25 Minutes
Servings: 5

Ingredients

- 2 tablespoons sesame oil
- 1 onion, chopped
- 2 bell peppers, chopped
- 1 parsnip, trimmed and chopped
- 1 carrot, trimmed and chopped
- 1 cup broccoli florets
- 2 garlic cloves, finely chopped
- 1/2 teaspoon ground cumin
- 2 cups brown rice
- Sea salt and black pepper, to taste
- 1/2 teaspoon ground turmeric
- 2 tablespoons fresh cilantro, finely chopped

Instructions

1. Heat the sesame oil in a saucepan over medium-high heat.
2. Once hot, cook the onion, peppers, parsnip, carrot, and broccoli for about 3 minutes until aromatic.
3. Add in the garlic and ground cumin; continue to cook for 30 seconds more until aromatic.
4. Place the brown rice in a saucepan and cover with cold water by 2 inches. Bring to a boil. Turn the heat to a simmer and continue to cook for about 30 minutes or until tender.
5. Stir the rice into the vegetable mixture; season with salt, black pepper, and ground turmeric; garnish with fresh cilantro and serve immediately. Bon appétit!

Nutrition Information

Calories: 363; Fat: 7.5g; Carbohydrates: 66.3g; Protein: 7.7g

Old Fashion Pilaf

Preparation Time: 5 Minutes
Cooking Time: 40 Minutes
Servings: 4

Ingredients

- 2 tablespoons sesame oil
- 1 shallot, sliced
- 2 bell peppers, seeded and sliced
- 3 cloves garlic, minced
- 10 ounces oyster mushrooms, cleaned and sliced
- 2 cups brown rice
- 2 tomatoes, pureed
- 2 cups vegetable broth
- Salt and black pepper, to taste
- 1 cup sweet corn kernels
- 1 cup green peas

Instructions

1. Heat the sesame oil in a saucepan over medium-high heat.
2. Once hot, cook the shallot and peppers for about 3 minutes until just tender.
3. Add in the garlic and oyster mushrooms; continue to sauté for 1 minute or so until aromatic.
4. In a lightly oiled casserole dish, place the rice, flowed by the mushroom mixture, tomatoes, broth, salt, black pepper, corn, and green peas.
5. Bake, covered, at 375 degrees F for about 40 minutes, stirring after 20 minutes. Bon appétit!

Nutrition Information

Calories: 532; Fat: 11.4g; Carbohydrates: 93g; Protein: 16.32g

Polenta with Mushrooms and Chickpeas

Preparation Time: 10 Minutes

Cooking Time: 25 minutes

Servings: 4

Ingredients

- 3 cups vegetable broth
- 1 cup yellow cornmeal
- 2 tablespoons olive oil
- 1 onion, chopped
- 1 bell pepper, seeded and sliced
- 1 pound Cremini mushrooms, sliced
- 2 garlic cloves, minced
- 1/2 cup dry white wine
- 1/2 cup vegetable broth
- Kosher salt and freshly ground black pepper, to taste
- 1 teaspoon paprika
- 1 cup canned chickpeas, drained

Instructions

1. In a medium saucepan, bring the vegetable broth to a boil over medium-high heat. Now, add in the cornmeal, whisking continuously to prevent lumps.

2. Reduce the heat to a simmer. Continue to simmer, whisking periodically, for about 18 minutes, until the mixture has thickened.

3. Meanwhile, heat the olive oil in a saucepan over a moderately high heat. Cook the onion and pepper for about 3 minutes or until just tender and fragrant.

4. Add in the mushrooms and garlic; continue to sauté, gradually adding the wine and broth, for 4 more minutes or until cooked through. Season with salt, black pepper and paprika. Stir in the chickpeas.

5. Spoon the mushroom mixture over your polenta and serve warm. Bon appétit!

Nutrition Information

Calories:488; Fat: 12.2g; Carbohydrates: 71g; Protein: 21.5g

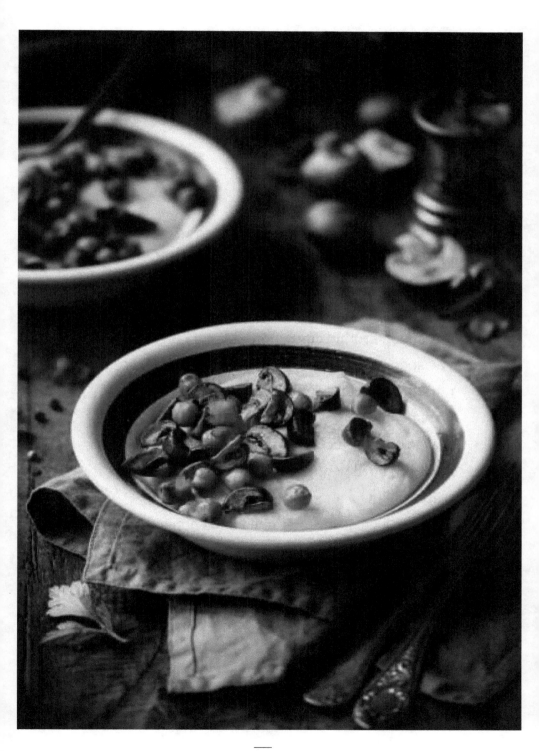

Preparation Time: 10 Minutes

Cooking Time: 15 minutes

Servings: 2

Ingredients

- 1 (8-ounce) package tempeh, cut into 16 cubes
- 1 tablespoon minced garlic
- 1 tablespoon unseasoned rice vinegar
- 1 tablespoon low-sodium soy sauce or tamari
- 1 teaspoon ground cinnamon
- 1 teaspoon ground turmeric
- 1 teaspoon ground cumin
- 1 teaspoon chili powder
- 2 large carrots, diced
- 1 large red bell pepper, seeded and sliced
- 1 large yellow bell pepper, seeded and sliced
- 6 ounces kale, leaves stemmed and chopped
- 2 teaspoons arrowroot powder

Instructions

1. Place the tempeh in a medium bowl. Set aside.

2. In a small bowl, combine the garlic, vinegar, soy sauce, cinnamon, turmeric, cumin, and chili powder and whisk until combined. Pour the mixture over the tempeh and let sit for 5 minutes.

3. Drain the tempeh, reserving the marinade.

4. In a large skillet or wok, cook the tempeh over medium heat, stirring, until it begins to brown, 4 to 6 minutes. Add the carrots, bell peppers, and kale and cook, stirring, until the kale has brightened in color and the carrots are tender, 3 to 5 minutes.

5. Whisk the arrowroot into the reserved marinade until smooth. Pour the mixture into the skillet, stir to combine, and simmer for just 3 minutes more.

6. Divide the tempeh mixture between two plates, drizzle with the thickened marinade, and serve.

Nutrition Information

Calories: 378; Fat: 3g; Protein: 28g; Carbohydrates: 43g

Cauliflower, Navy Beans and Quinoa Risotto

Preparation Time: 15 Minutes
Cooking Time: 45 minutes
Servings: 4

Ingredients

- 5 to 6 cups cauliflower, cut into 1- to 1½-inch florets
- Salt, to taste (optional)
- Ground black or white pepper, to taste
- 2 cups cooked navy beans
- 2 ⅓ cups low-sodium vegetable broth, divided
- 1 tablespoon fresh lemon juice
- Pinch of nutritional yeast
- 4 to 5 shallots, finely diced
- 2 teaspoons minced fresh thyme leaves (about 4 sprigs)
- 1 cup quinoa
- ½ cup chopped fresh flat-leaf parsley

Instructions

1. Preheat the oven to 400°F (205°C). Line a baking sheet with parchment paper.
2. Arrange the cauliflower florets on the baking sheet. Sprinkle with salt (if desired) and pepper. Toss to coat well.
3. Roast in the preheated oven for 25 minutes or until golden brown. Flip the florets every 5 minutes to roast evenly.
4. Meanwhile, put the navy beans, 1/3 cup of the vegetable broth, lemon juice, and nutritional yeast in a food processor. Pulse to purée until creamy and smooth. Set aside.
5. Heat a saucepan over medium heat. Add the shallots and sauté for 4 minutes or until lightly browned.
6. Add the thyme to the pan and sauté for 1 minute or until aromatic.
7. Make the risotto: Add the quinoa and remaining vegetable broth to the pan. Stir to combine well. Bring to a boil, then reduce the heat to medium-low and simmer for 14 minutes or until the liquid is mostly absorbed.
8. Mix in the navy bean purée. Sprinkle with salt (if desired) and pepper. Spread the parsley and roasted cauliflower florets over the risotto. Serve warm.

Nutrition Information

Calories: 456; Fat: 5.1g Carbohydrates: 84.9g; Protein: 21.7g

Butternut Squash with Quinoa and Almonds

Preparation Time: 20 Minutes

Cooking Time: 25-30 Minutes

Servings: 4

Ingredients

- 1 medium (1½-pound/680-g) butternut squash, deseeded and cut into 1-inch cubes
- ¼ teaspoon dried chili flakes
- 1 teaspoon smoked paprika
- 1 clove garlic, thinly sliced
- 1 teaspoon fresh thyme leaves (about 2 sprigs)
- Salt, to taste (optional)
- Ground black or white pepper, to taste
- 12 green olives
- 4 lemon slices
    Almond Quinoa:
- ¾ cup cooked quinoa
- 1/3 cup chopped arugula
- 1/3 cup chopped fresh flat-leaf parsley
- 1 teaspoon fresh lemon juice
- Salt, to taste (optional)
- Ground black or white pepper, to taste
- ¼ cup toasted and chopped almonds

Instructions

1. Preheat the oven to 400°F (205°C). Line a baking sheet with a parchment paper.
2. Combine the butternut squash with chili flakes, paprika, garlic, thyme, salt (if desired), and pepper in a large bowl. Toss to coat well.
3. Pour the butternut squash mixture in the baking sheet, then top them with olives and lemon slices.
4. Bake in the preheated oven for 25 to 30 minutes or until the butternut squash cubes are soft. Shake the baking sheet every 5 or 10 minutes so the cubes are cooked evenly.
5. Meanwhile, combine the cooked quinoa with arugula, parsley, lemon juice, salt (if desired), and pepper on a large serving plate. Toss to combine well.
6. Top the quinoa with cooked butternut squash and almond before serving

Nutrition Information

Calories: 172; Fat: 5.1g; Carbohydrates: 30.2g; Protein: 5.2g

Preparation Time: 50 Minutes

Cooking Time: 6-10 Minutes

Servings: 4

Ingredients

- 3 tablespoons cumin seeds
- 3 tablespoons caraway seeds
- 3 tablespoons coriander seeds
- 2 tablespoons tomato paste
- 1/3 cup fresh lemon juice
- 1 tablespoon lemon zest
- 2 cloves garlic, chopped
- 3 to 4 small red chili peppers, seeded and chopped
- Salt, to taste (optional)
- Ground black or white pepper, to taste
- 2 tablespoons low-sodium vegetable broth
- 1 cup cooked French or black beluga lentils
  Cauliflower Rice:
- 6 cups chopped cauliflower florets
- 1 tablespoon low-sodium vegetable broth
- Salt, to taste (optional)
- Ground black or white pepper, to taste
- ¼ cup chopped fresh mint leaves
- ¼ cup chopped fresh flat-leaf parsley
- 2 teaspoons fresh lemon juice
- 2 green onions, thinly sliced

Instructions

1. Heat a skillet over medium heat, then add and sauté the seeds to toast for 2 minutes or until lightly browned.

2. Make the harissa: Pour the toasted seeds in a food processor, then add the tomato paste, lemon juice and zest, garlic, chili peppers, salt (if desired), and pepper. Process until the mixture is creamy and smooth. Pour the harissa in a bowl and set aside until ready to use.

3. Heat the vegetable broth in a saucepan over medium heat. Add the cooked lentils and ¾ cup of harissa to the pan and simmer for 5 to 10 minutes until the mixture is glossy and smooth and has a thick consistency. Keep stirring during the simmering.

4. Put the cauliflower florets in a food processor, then process to rice the cauliflower.

5. Heat the vegetable broth in a nonstick skillet over medium heat. Add the riced cauliflower, then sprinkle with salt (if desired) and pepper. Sauté for 1 minute or until lightly softened.

6. Transfer the cooked cauliflower rice to a large bowl, then add the mint, parsley, lemon juice, and green onions. Toss to combine well.

7. Serve the riced cauliflower with harissa lentils on top.

Nutrition Information

Calories: 176; Protein: 11.2g; Carbohydrates: 32.2g; Fats: 3.4g

Preparation Time: 40 Minutes
Cooking Time: 30 Minutes
Servings: 6 pancakes

Ingredients

- 1 cup semi-pearled farro
- ¼ cup toasted and chopped pine nuts
- 1 teaspoon nutritional yeast
- 1 tablespoon fresh lemon juice
- 1 teaspoon lemon zest
- Salt, to taste (optional)
- Ground black or white pepper, to taste
- 8 chard leaves
- 2 cups low-sodium marinara sauce
- ½ cup water

Instructions

1. Preheat the oven to 350°F (180°C).

2. Combine the cooked farro, pine nuts, nutritional yeast, lemon juice and zest, salt (if desired), and pepper in a mixing bowl. Set aside.

3. Remove the stems of the chard leaves so you have 16 chard leaf halves, then blanch the leaves in a bowl of boiling water for 5 minutes or until wilted.

4. Pour ½ cup of marinara sauce on a baking dish. Take a chard half, then spoon 2 tablespoons of farro mixture in the middle of the leaf half. Fold the leaf over the filling, then tuck the leaf and roll up to wrap the filling. Repeat with remaining chard and farro mixture.

5. Arrange the chard rolls on the baking dish over the marinara sauce, seam side down, then top them with remaining marinara sauce and water.

6. Cover the baking dish with aluminum foil and bake in the preheated oven for 30 minutes or until the sauce bubbles.

7. Remove the chard rolls from the oven and serve immediately.

Nutrition Information

Calories: 254; Fats: 9g; Carbohydrates: 39g; Protein: 7.7g

Rice with Almonds, Parsley and Cranberries

Preparation Time: 10 Minutes
Cooking Time: 40 Minutes
Servings: 2
Ingredients

- 1 cup wild and brown rice blend, rinsed
- ¼ teaspoon ground sumac
- ¼ cup chopped almonds, for garnish
- ¼ cup chopped fresh flat-leaf parsley
- ¼ cup unsweetened dried cranberries
- ½ teaspoon ground coriander
- 1 teaspoon apple cider vinegar
- 2 green onions, thinly sliced
- Salt, to taste (optional)
- Ground black or white pepper, to taste

Instructions

1. Pour the rice blend in a saucepan, then pour in the water to cover the rice by about 1 inch. Bring to a boil over medium-high heat. Reduce the heat to low. Put the pan lid on and simmer for 40 minutes or until the water is absorbed. Transfer the rice to a bowl and allow to cool for 5 minutes.

2. Add the remaining ingredient to the bowl and toss to combine well. Serve immediately.

Nutrition Information

Calories: 105g; Fat: 0.9g; Carbohydrates: 21.1g; Protein: 3.1g

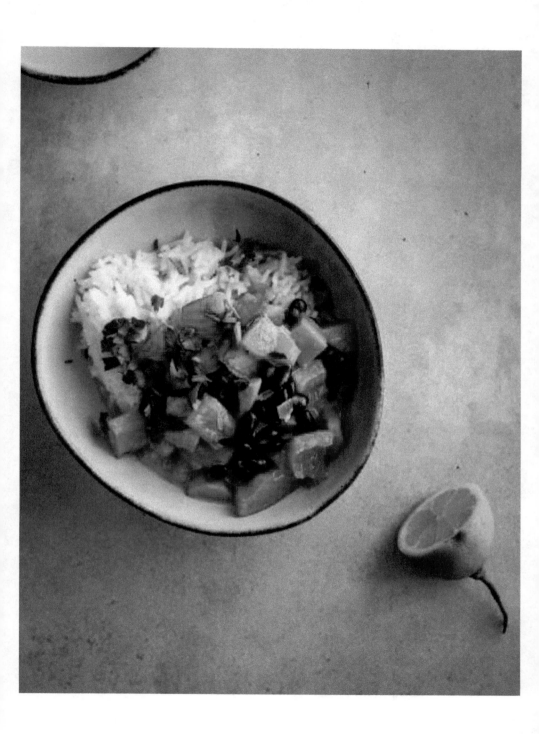

Dinner

Simple Pizza Recipe

Preparation Time: 10 Minutes

Cooking Time: 15 Minutes

Total Time: 25 Minutes

Serves: 6-8

Ingredients

- 1 pizza crust -
- ½ cup tomato sauce -
- ¼ black pepper -
- 1 cup pepperoni slices -
- 1 cup mozzarella cheese -
- 1 cup olives

Instructions

1. Spread tomato sauce on the pizza crust
2. Place all the toppings on the pizza crust
3. Bake the pizza at 425 F for 12-15 minutes
4. When ready remove pizza from the oven and serve

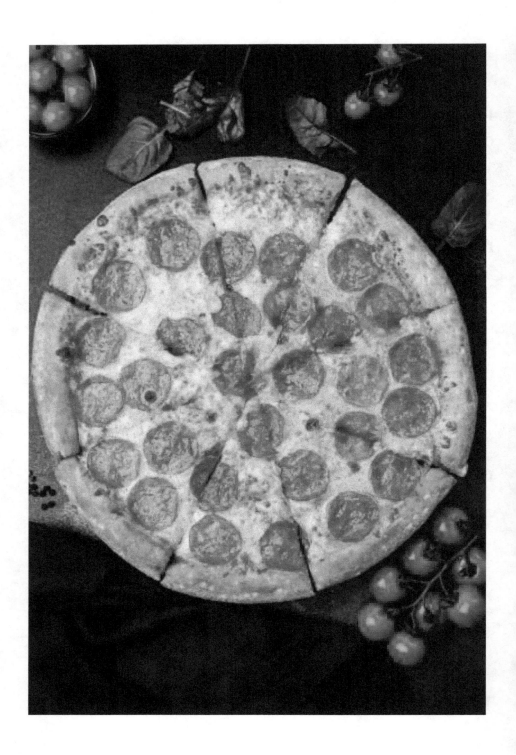

Red Onion Frittata

Preparation Time: 10 Minutes

Cooking Time: 20 Minutes

Total Time: 30 Minutes

Serves: 2

Ingredients

- ½ lb. asparagus -
- 1 tablespoon olive oil -
- ½ red onion -
- ¼ tsp salt -
- 2 eggs -
- 2 oz. cheddar cheese -
- 1 garlic clove -
- ¼ tsp dill

Instructions

1. In a bowl whisk eggs with salt and cheese
2. In a frying pan heat olive oil and pour egg mixture
3. Add remaining ingredients and mix well
4. Serve when ready

Tomato and Onion Pasta

Preparation Time: 10 Minutes

Cooking Time: 20 Minutes

Total Time: 30 Minutes

Serves: 2

Ingredients

- 1 tablespoon olive oil -
- 1 onion -
- ½ lb. penne pasta -
- 2-3 garlic cloves -
- 1 oz. parsley -
- ½ lb. tomatoes -
- ¼ lb. low fat sour cream

Instructions

1. Heat olive oil in a pan and sauté onion until soft
2. Add pasta, garlic, pasta, and water to cover
3. Bring to a boil and simmer for 5-6 minutes
4. Add tomatoes and cook for another 4-5 minutes
5. Drain the pasta mixture and return to the pan
6. Stir in soured cream
7. Garnish with parsley and serve

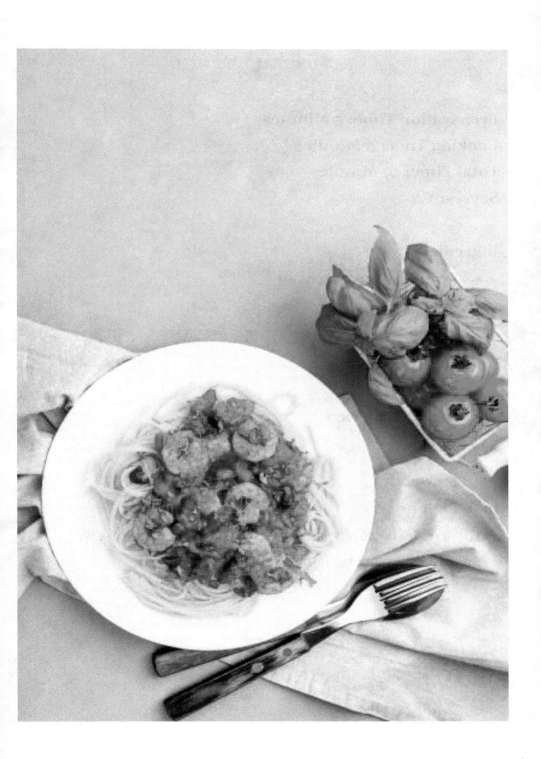

Couscous Salad

Preparation Time: 5 Minutes
Cooking Time: 5 Minutes
Total Time: 10 Minutes
Serves: 1

Ingredients

- 1 cup cooked couscous -
- ¼ cup pine nuts -
- 1 shallot -
- 2 cloves garlic -
- 1 can chickpeas -
- 2 oz. low fat cheese -
- 1 zucchini

Instructions

1. In a bowl combine all ingredients together and mix well
2. Add salad dressing, toss well, and serve

Broccoli Frittata

Preparation Time: 10 Minutes
Cooking Time: 20 Minutes
Total Time: 30 Minutes
Serves: 2

Ingredients

- 1 cup broccoli -
- 1 tablespoon olive oil -
- ½ red onion -
- 2 eggs -
- ¼ tsp salt -
- 2 oz. cheddar cheese -
- 1 garlic clove -
- ¼ tsp dill

Instructions

1. In a bowl whisk eggs with salt and cheese
2. In a frying pan heat olive oil and pour egg mixture
3. Add remaining ingredients and mix well
4. Serve when ready

Cauliflower & Farro Salad

Preparation Time: 5 Minutes

Cooking Time: 5 Minutes

Total Time: 10 Minutes

Serves: 1

Ingredients

- 1 cauliflower -
- 1 tablespoon olive oil -
- ¼ tsp black pepper -
- 1 cup cooked Farro -
- 2 garlic cloves -
- ¼ cup feta cheese -
- 1 avocado

Instructions

1. In a bowl combine all ingredients together and mix well
2. Add salad dressing, toss well, and serve

Cheese Macaroni

Preparation Time: 10 Minutes
Cooking Time: 20 Minutes
Total Time: 30 Minutes
Serves: 1

Ingredients

- 1 lb. macaroni -
- 1 cup cheddar cheese -
- 1 cup Monterey Jack cheese -
- 1 cup mozzarella cheese -
- ¼ tsp salt -
- ¼ tsp pepper

Instructions

1. In a pot bring water to a boil
2. Add pasta and cook until al dente
3. In a bowl combine all cheese together and add it to the pasta
4. When ready transfer to a bowl, add salt, pepper, and serve

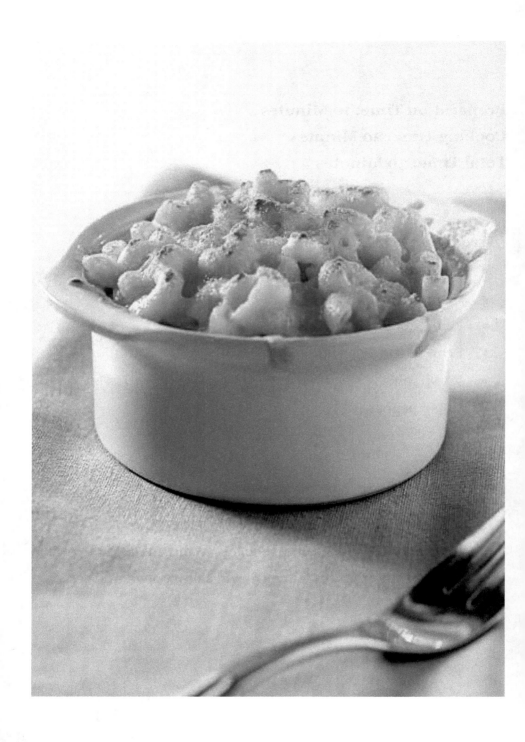

Entrée

Grilled Lobster with Garlic-Parsley Butter (Griddle Pan)

Preparation Time: 10 minutes

Cooking Time: 10 Minutes

Serves: 2 Servings (1 lobster half per serving)

Ingredients

- 1 lobster, about 1 ½ pound
- 2 teaspoons minced garlic
- 1 lemon, zested
- 1 teaspoon salt
- 1 ½ teaspoon crushed red chili flakes
- ½ teaspoon ground black pepper
- 2 tablespoons chopped parsley
- ¼ cup olive oil
- 8 tablespoons butter, unsalted, softened

Instructions

1. Using a medium bowl, place parsley, garlic, and butter in it. Add salt, black pepper, lemon zest, parsley, and red chili flakes. Then stir until combined, set aside until needed.

2. Set up the grill and set it to a high-heat setting. Preheat. A large griddle pan can also be used.

3. Meanwhile, prepare the lobster, split it in half lengthwise from head to tail by using a cleaver. Break off its claws, and then discard its green-yellow tomalley.

4. Place lobster halves on a large baking sheet, shell-side down along with claws. Drizzle with oil, and then season with salt, and black pepper.

5. Place the prepared lobster halves flesh-side-down and claws on the grill, and then cook for 3 minutes until slightly charred.

6. Carefully turn the lobster meat and spread the prepared garlic-parsley mixture over it and continue grilling for 5 minutes.

7. Serve right away.

Nutrition Information Per Serving:

Carbohydrates: 1.7 grams/Fat: 72.4 grams/Protein: 14.1 grams/Fiber: 0 grams/Calories: 708

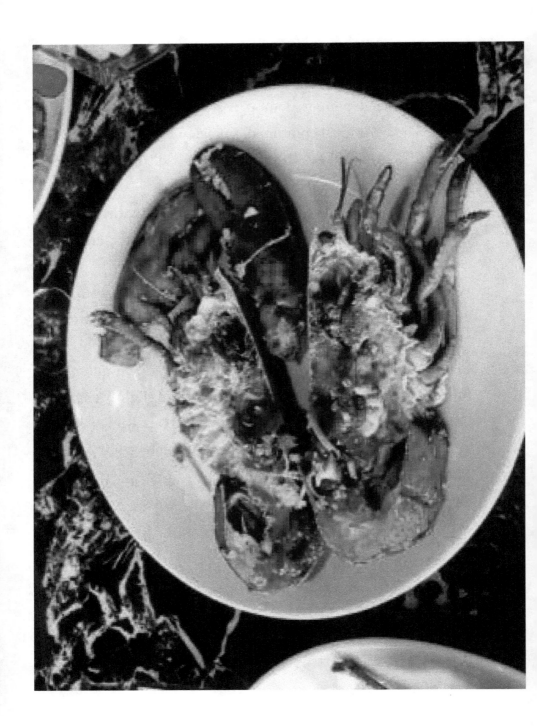

Marinated Mackerel (Griddle Pan)

Preparation Time: 25 minutes
Cooking Time: 12 Minutes
Serves: 4 Servings (1 fillet)

Ingredients

- 4 fillets of mackerel, with skin, each about 4 to 6 ounces
- 1 teaspoon salt
- 1 teaspoon ground black pepper
- Non-stick cooking oil spray

For the Marinade:

- ½ tablespoon grated ginger
- ½ tablespoon minced garlic
- 3 tablespoons soy sauce
- 2 tablespoons olive oil
- 1 lemon, juiced

Instructions

1. Using a large bowl, place all the ingredients to be marinated. Stir until well blended.

2. Add mackerel fillets and toss until coated. Cover the bowl, and then let the fish marinate for a minimum of 20 minutes.

3. Get a griddle pan. Grease it with oil and place over medium-high heat.

4. Arrange the marinated fish fillets on the griddle pan (skin-side up) and cook for 5 minutes.

5. Turn the fish fillets, and drizzle with the remaining marinade. Season with salt, and black pepper. Continue cooking for 5 to 7 minutes until fillets have thoroughly cooked.

6. Serve right away or serve with boiled rice.

Nutrition Information Per Serving:

Carbohydrates: 0.8 grams/Fat: 26.7 grams/Protein: 20.3 grams/Fiber: 0.1 grams/Calories: 326

Mackerel Fish Fry (Air Fryer)

Preparation Time: 25 minutes

Cooking Time: 12 Minutes

Serves: 5 Servings (1 fish per serving)

Ingredients

- 5 whole mackerel fish, gutted, cleaned
- 1 lemon, cut into wedges
- Non-stick cooking oil spray

For the Marinade:

- 1 teaspoon minced garlic
- ½ teaspoon grated ginger
- 3 sprigs of curry leaves, chopped
- 1 tablespoon red chili powder
- 1 teaspoon salt
- 1 teaspoon red chili flakes
- ½ teaspoon turmeric powder
- ½ teaspoon vinegar
- 3 tablespoons olive oil, melted

Instructions

1. Prepare the fish. Remove its inside, rinse well until cleaned, and pat dry. Make 3 to 4 small cuts on each fish.

2. Using a small bowl, place all the ingredients to be marinated, and stir until well combined.

3. Brush the marinade on all sides of each fish. Make sure it goes into the cut and the fish is evenly seasoned. Marinate the fish for a minimum of 20 minutes in the refrigerator.

4. When ready to cook, switch on the air fryer, and grease its frying basket with oil. Insert it into the fryer and close the cover. Select the cooking temperature up to 400 degrees F and preheat.

5. Arrange the marinated fish in a single layer, and place in the fryer's basket. Set the frying time to 12 minutes, and then let it cook until fork tender.

6. When done, transfer the fish to a plate and then serve with lemon wedges.

Nutrition Information Per Serving:

Carbohydrates: 1.3 grams/Fat: 42.8 grams/Protein: 30.8 grams/Fiber: 0.02 grams/Calories: 515

Fried Crumbed Mackerel (Air Fryer)

Preparation Time: 10 minutes
Cooking Time: 12 Minutes
Serves: 4 Servings (1 fish per serving)

Ingredients

- 4 mackerel fish, gutted, cleaned
- ¾ cup breadcrumbs
- ½ cup tempura flour
- ½ teaspoon garlic powder
- ½ teaspoon salt
- ½ cup of water
- Non-stick cooking oil spray

Instructions

1. Prepare the mackerel fish. Remove its head, tail, and insides. Rinse well until clean, and then pat dry.
2. Cut the fish into bite-size pieces. Place in a large bowl, season with salt and garlic powder Then toss until coated.
3. Take a separate bowl, and place tempura flour in it. Whisk in water until smooth batter comes together, and let it rest for 15 minutes.
4. Spread breadcrumbs in a shallow dish.
5. Switch on the air fryer and grease its frying basket with oil. Insert it into the fryer and close the cover. Select the cooking temperature up to 400 degrees F and preheat.
6. Work on one fish piece at a time. Dip the fish into the tempura flour mixture, and then lightly coat in breadcrumbs until all side are covered.
7. Then arrange the prepared fish pieces in a single layer. Place them in the fryer's basket. Set the frying time to 12 minutes, and let it cook until crispy, turning halfway and spraying with oil.
8. When done, transfer fried mackerel to a plate, and then serve with chili sauce.

Nutrition Information Per Serving:

Carbohydrates: 27.5 grams/Fat: 45.8 grams/Protein: 43 grams/Fiber: 1.4 grams/Calories: 690

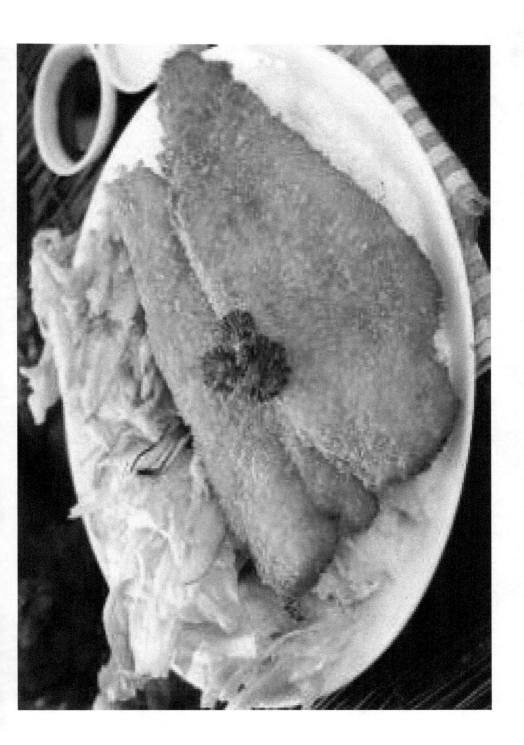

Fried Mackerel with Ginger Sauce (Pan)

Preparation Time: 20 minutes

Cooking Time: 12 Minutes

Serves: 2 Servings (1 fillet per serving)

Ingredients

- 2 fillets of Mackerel, skin on, each about 4 to 6 ounces
- 1 teaspoon salt
- 2 tablespoons olive oil

For the Sauce:

- 2 teaspoons chopped garlic
- ¼ teaspoon sugar
- 3 teaspoons chopped ginger
- 1 tablespoon corn starch
- 1 teaspoon oyster sauce
- ½ cup and 2 tablespoons water, divided
- 1 teaspoon soy sauce

Instructions

1. Rinse the fillets, and pat dry. Place them on a cutting board (skin-side up). Make a criss-cross pattern on the flesh.
2. Cut each fillet in half, season with salt until coated on all sides. Let the fillets rest for 15 minutes.
3. Using a large frying pan, place it over medium heat and add oil.
4. Add fish fillet, and cook for 3 to 4 minutes per side, or until fork tender. Then transfer to a plate.
5. Prepare the sauce by adding ginger and garlic. Cook for 1 minute until fragrant.
6. Pour in ½ cup water, soy sauce, sugar, and oyster sauce, and then stir until well mixed.
7. Get a small bowl, add cornstarch, and stir in remaining water until smooth. Place the mixture in a frying pan.
8. Cook the sauce for 2 to 3 minutes until thickened to the desired level, and then pour into a serving bowl.
9. Serve the sauce with fish fillets.

Nutrition Information Per Serving:

Carbohydrates: 6 grams/Fat: 33.4 grams/Protein: 20.3 grams/Fiber: 0.2 grams/Calories: 406

Teriyaki Mackerel (Air Fryer)

Preparation Time: 5 minutes

Cooking Time: 25 Minutes

Serves: 5 Servings (1/2-pound fillets per serving)

Ingredients

- 1½ lbs mackerel fillets, skin on
- 2 green onions, sliced
- Non-stick cooking oil spray

For the Teriyaki sauce:

- ½ teaspoon minced garlic
- ½ cup maple syrup or honey
- 2 teaspoons chopped ginger
- 1 cup of soy sauce
- 1 lemon, zested
- 1 cup of rice wine

Instructions

1. Place a medium saucepan over medium heat, then add all the ingredients for the sauce. Stir until well combined.

2. Bring the sauce to a boil, and switch heat to medium-low level. Let it simmer for 15 to 20 minutes until reduced by half. Uncover the pan and when done, strain the sauce.

3. Switch on the air fryer and grease its frying basket with oil. Insert it into the fryer and close the cover. Select the cooking temperature up to 400 degrees F and preheat.

4. Brush the fish fillets with the prepared teriyaki sauce. Arrange the fillets into the fryer basket (skin-side down). Set the frying time to 5 minutes, and then let it cook.

5. After 5 minutes, turn the fillets, and brush with the teriyaki sauce. Continue frying for 5 minutes until fillets have turned fork tender.

6. When done, transfer fish fillets to a plate, and drizzle with remaining teriyaki sauce. Sprinkle with green onions, and then serve.

Nutrition Information Per Serving:

Carbohydrates: 24 grams/Fat: 29.7 grams/Protein: 28.6 grams/Fiber: 0.8 grams/Calories: 478

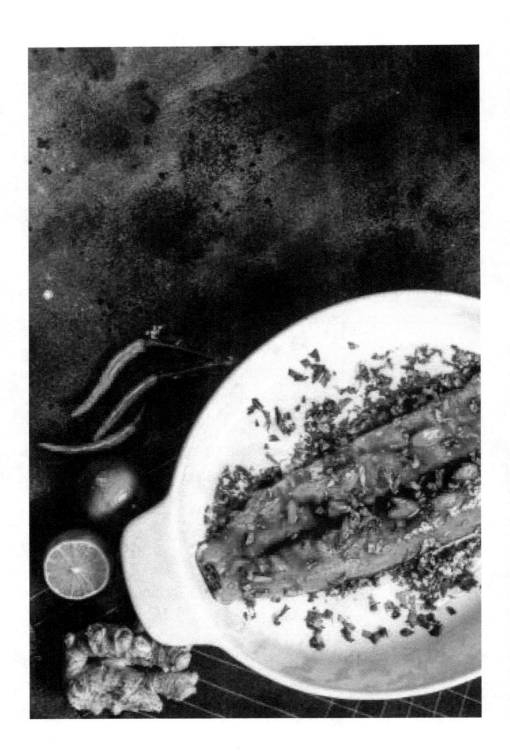

Honey Soy Mackerel (Air Fryer)

Preparation Time: 30 minutes

Cooking Time: 10 Minutes

Serves: 4 Servings (1 fillet per serving)

Ingredients

- 4 whole mackerel, gutted, cleaned

For the Marinade:

- 1 red chili, chopped
- 1 lime, juiced, zested
- 1 teaspoon minced garlic
- 1 teaspoon honey
- 2 tablespoons soy sauce
- 4 tablespoons olive oil
- 1 tablespoon sesame oil

Instructions

1. Place all the ingredients for the marinade in a large bowl, and whisk until combined.

2. Prepare the mackerel. Remove its head, tail, and insides. Rinse well until clean, and pat dry.

3. Add the fish into the prepared marinade and toss until well coated. Cover the bowl with its lid, and then let the fish marinate for a minimum of 20 minutes at room temperature.

4. Switch on the air fryer. Grease its frying basket with oil and insert it into the fryer. Close the cover and select the cooking temperature up to 400 degrees F and preheat.

5. Arrange the marinated fish in a single layer, and place in the fryer's basket. Set the frying time to 10 minutes, and let it cook until fork-tender, turning halfway and spraying with oil.

6. Serve right away.

Nutrition Information Per Serving:

Carbohydrates: 4.2 grams/Fat: 46.8 grams/Protein: 30.8 grams/Fiber: 0.7 grams/Calories: 562

Blackened Mullet (Air Fryer)

Preparation Time: 10 minutes

Cooking Time: 10 Minutes

Serves: 6 Servings (1/2 pound per serving)

Ingredients

- 3 pounds mullet fillets, skinless
- ¼ cup butter, unsalted, melted
- Non-stick cooking oil spray

The Spice Mix:

- ½ tablespoon garlic powder
- ½ tablespoon onion powder
- ½ teaspoon ground black pepper
- ½ teaspoon mustard powder
- ½ teaspoon cayenne pepper
- ¾ teaspoon salt
- ½ teaspoon dried thyme
- ½ tablespoon sweet paprika

Instructions

1. Using a small bowl, place all the ingredients for the spice mix, and then stir until well blended.

2. Switch on the air fryer and grease its frying basket with oil. Insert it into the fryer and close the cover. Select the cooking temperature up to 400 degrees F and preheat.

3. Meanwhile, brush the fillets with melted butter, and sprinkle with the prepared spice mix until well coated.

4. Arrange the prepared fillets in a single layer, and place in the fryer's basket. Set the frying time to 10 minutes, and then let it cook until fork-tender, turning halfway and spraying with oil.

5. Serve immediately.

Nutrition Information Per Serving:

Carbohydrates: 1.2 grams/Fat: 22.4 grams/Protein: 60.4 grams/Fiber: 0.2 grams/Calories: 449

Mullet with Garlic Oil (Air Fryer)

Preparation Time: 10 minutes

Cooking Time: 10 Minutes

Serves: 4 Servings (4 fillets per serving)

Ingredients

- 4 whole mullets, gutted, cleaned
- 2 teaspoons salt
- 2 teaspoon ground black pepper
- Non-stick cooking oil spray

For the Garlic Oil:

- 2 fillets of anchovy
- 3 cloves of garlic, peeled, chopped
- ½ tablespoon red chili flakes
- 1 tablespoon parsley leaves, chopped
- 2 tablespoons sunflower oil
- 1/3 cup olive oil

Instructions

1. Switch on the air fryer and grease its frying basket with oil. Insert it into the fryer and close the cover. Select the cooking temperature up to 400 degrees F and preheat.

2. Prepare the fillet. Season with salt, and black pepper.

3. Arrange the prepared fillets in a single layer in the fryer's basket. Set the frying time to 10 minutes, and then let it cook until fork-tender, turning halfway and spraying with oil.

4. While still frying the fish, prepare the garlic oil. Use a small saucepan and place it over medium heat. Add chili flakes, anchovy, and sunflower oil.

5. Stir until well combined. Cook for 7 to 10 minutes until anchovy melts. Remove the pan from heat. Add olive oil, stir until mixed and let it cool until needed.

6. Stir parsley into the garlic oil. Scoop it evenly on four plates and add a fried fillet to each, and then serve.

Nutrition Information Per Serving:

Carbohydrates: 1.5 grams/Fat: 41.5 grams/Protein: 55.8 grams/Fiber: 0.05 grams/Calories: 605

Smoothie

Peanut Butter Smoothie

Preparation Time: 5 Minutes
Cooking Time: 5 Minutes
Total Time: 10 Minutes
Serves: 2

Ingredients

- 1 cup milk -
- 1 large banana -
- 3 tablespoons peanut butter

Instructions

1. In a blender place all ingredients and blend until smooth
2. Pour smoothie in a glass and serve

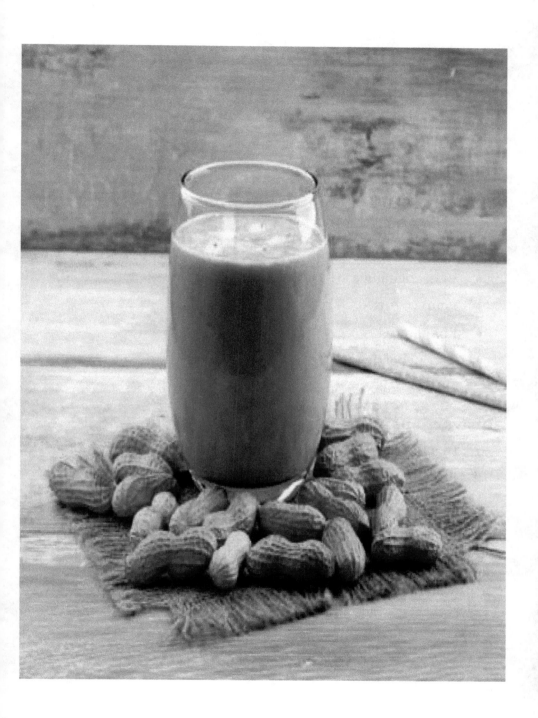

Strawberry Smoothie

Preparation Time: 5 Minutes

Cooking Time: 5 Minutes

Total Time: 10 Minutes

Serves: 1

Ingredients

- ¼ orange juice -
- 1 cup yogurt -
- 1 banana -
- 4 strawberries

Instructions

1. In a blender place all ingredients and blend until smooth
2. Pour smoothie in a glass and serve

Avocado Smoothie

Preparation Time: 5 Minutes

Cooking Time: 5 Minutes

Total Time: 10 Minutes

Serves: 2

Ingredients

- 1 cup milk -
- ½ avocado -
- 1 banana

Instructions

1. In a blender place all ingredients and blend until smooth
2. Pour smoothie in a glass and serve

Watermelon Smoothie

Preparation Time: 5 Minutes

Cooking Time: 5 Minutes

Total Time: 10 Minutes

Serves: 1

Ingredients

- 2 cups watermelon -
- 1 cup almond milk -
- 1 cup vanilla yogurt -
- 2 tablespoons maple syrup -
- 1 cup ice

Instructions

1. In a blender place all ingredients and blend until smooth
2. Pour smoothie in a glass and serve

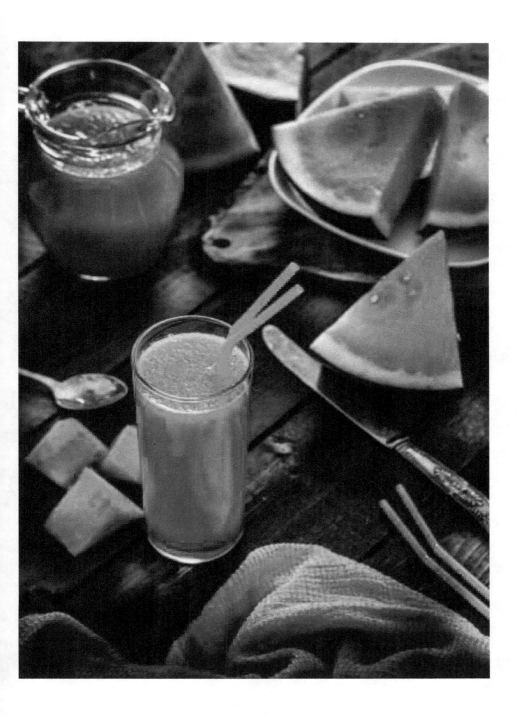

Strawberry Banana Smoothie

Preparation Time: 5 Minutes
Cooking Time: 5 Minutes
Total Time: 10 Minutes
Serves: 1

Ingredients

- 1 cup raspberries -
- 1 cup strawberries -
- 1 banana -
- 1 cup almond milk -
- 1 tablespoon honey -
- 1 cup ice

Instructions

1. In a blender place all ingredients and blend until smooth
2. Pour smoothie in a glass and serve

Spinach Smoothie

Preparation Time: 5 Minutes
Cooking Time: 5 Minutes
Total Time: 10 Minutes
Serves: 1

Ingredients

- 2 cups banana -
- 2 cups strawberries -
- 2 cups spinach -
- 2 chia seeds

Instructions

1. In a blender place all ingredients and blend until smooth
2. Pour smoothie in a glass and serve

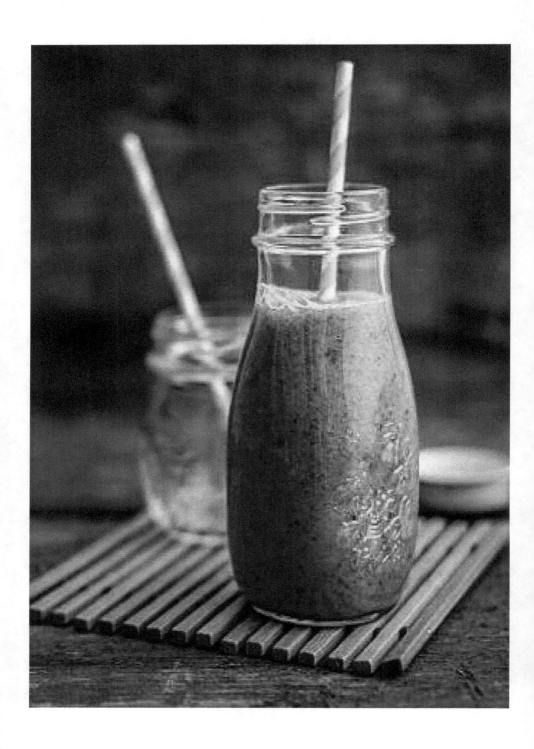

The Alkaline Strawberry Smoothie

Preparation Time: 5 minutes

Cooking Time: Nil

Serving: 2

Ingredients

- ½ cup of organic strawberries/blueberries
- Half a banana
- 2 cups of coconut water
- ½ inch ginger
- Juice of 2 grapefruits

Instructions

1. Add all the listed ingredients to a blender
2. Blend on high until smooth and creamy
3. Enjoy your smoothie

Nutrition Information (Per Serving)

Calories: 200 Fat: 10g Carbohydrates: 14g Protein 2g

Berry Smoothie

Preparation Time: 5 Minutes

Cooking Time: 0 Minutes

Servings: 2

Ingredients

- ½ cup of raspberries and blackberries
- 5 large strawberries
- 6 ounces of low-fat Greek yogurt
- 1 cup of crushed ice
- 1–2 drops of liquid stevia (optional)

Instructions

1. Add all ingredients into a food processor or a blender.
2. Blend well until smooth consistency.
3. Serve and enjoy

Nutrition Information

Calories: 76; Fat: 0.3g; Protein: 9g; Carbohydrates: 10g

Specials

Lobster Creole

Preparation Time: 20 minutes

Cooking Time: 40 minutes

Total Time: 60 Minutes

Serves: 10

Ingredients

- 6 lobster tails -
- 15 oz can crush tomatoes -
- 2 lb shrimp -
- 1/3 cup olive oil -
- 2 onions -
- 1 bunch Italian parley -
- 1 bay leaf -
- 1 cup ketchup -
- 2 tsp tabasco -
- 1 red pepper -
- 5 garlic cloves -
- 1 can pimentos -
- 2 tbs Worcestershire sauce -
- 5 oz tomato sauce -
- 1/3 cup wine -
- 2 tbs vinegar -
- Salt -
- Pepper

Instructions

1. Cut lobster tails into rings and sauté in hot oil until the shells turn red

2. Sauté the onion, garlic, red pepper, and bay leaf in the remaining oil for about 10 minutes

3. Stir in the Worcestershire sauce, tomato paste, wine, vinegar, parsley, crushed tomatoes, ketchup, and pimentos

4. Bring to a simmer and cook for 15 minutes, then season with salt and pepper

5. Return the lobster to the pot and simmer for at least 15 minutes

6. Stir in hot sauce Serve immediately

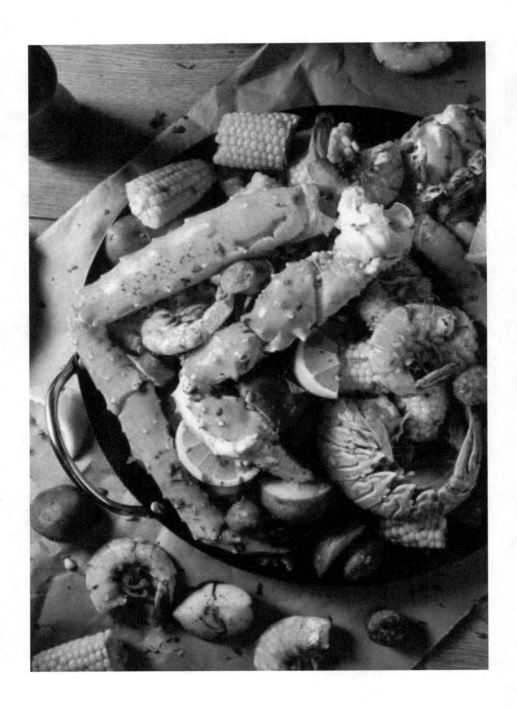

Grilled Salmon

Preparation Time: 5 Minutes

Cooking Time: 10 Minutes

Total Time: 15 Minutes

Serves: 4

Ingredients

- 2 limes juiced -
- 1 tbs cilantro -
- 1 ½ tsp cumin -
- 1 ½ tsp paprika -
- 2 lbs salmon -
- 1 ½ tbs oil -
- 1 tsp onion powder -
- 1 tsp chili powder -
- 1 avocado -
- 2 tsp salt -
- 1 red onion

Instructions

1. Mix the chili powder, onion powder, cumin, paprika, salt and pepper together
2. Rub the salmon with the mix and oil
3. Refrigerate for 30 minutes
4. Preheat the grill
5. Mix the avocado with lime juice, cilantro, and onion together
6. Grill the salmon
7. Serve topped with the avocado

Corn Pasta

Preparation Time: 5 Minutes
Cooking Time: 15 Minutes
Total Time: 20 Minutes
Serves: 2

Ingredients

- 1 lb. pasta -
- 4 oz. cheese -
- ¼ sour cream -
- 1 onion -
- 2 cloves garlic -
- 1 tsp cumin -
- 2 cups corn kernels -
- 1 tsp chili powder -
- 1 tablespoon cilantro

Instructions

1. In a pot boil spaghetti (or any other type of pasta), drain and set aside
2. Place all the ingredients for the sauce in a pot and bring to a simmer
3. Add pasta and mix well
4. When ready garnish with parmesan cheese and serve

Zucchini Soup

Preparation Time: 10 Minutes

Cooking Time: 20 Minutes

Total Time: 30 Minutes

Serves: 4

Ingredients

- 1 tablespoon olive oil -
- 1 lb. zucchini -
- ¼ red onion -
- ½ cup all-purpose flour -
- ¼ tsp salt -
- ¼ tsp pepper -
- 1 can vegetable broth -
- 1 cup heavy cream

Instructions

1. In a saucepan heat olive oil and sauté zucchini until tender
2. Add remaining ingredients to the saucepan and bring to a boil
3. When all the vegetables are tender transfer to a blender and blend until smooth
4. Pour soup into bowls, garnish with parsley and serve

Rosemary Lemon Tuna

Preparation Time: 130 Minutes

Cooking Time: 20 Minutes

Total Time: 150 Minutes

Serves: 4

Ingredients

- 3 cloves garlic -
- ½ cup lemon juice -
- 1 tsp salt -
- 3 tbs oil -
- 1 lb tuna -
- ½ cup rosemary

Instructions

1. Mix the lemon juice, oil, rosemary, salt, and garlic.
2. Rinse the tuna and pat dry. Place the tuna in a baking dish.
3. Pour the mixture over and refrigerate for 2-3 hours.
4. Grill the fish for 6 minutes on each side.

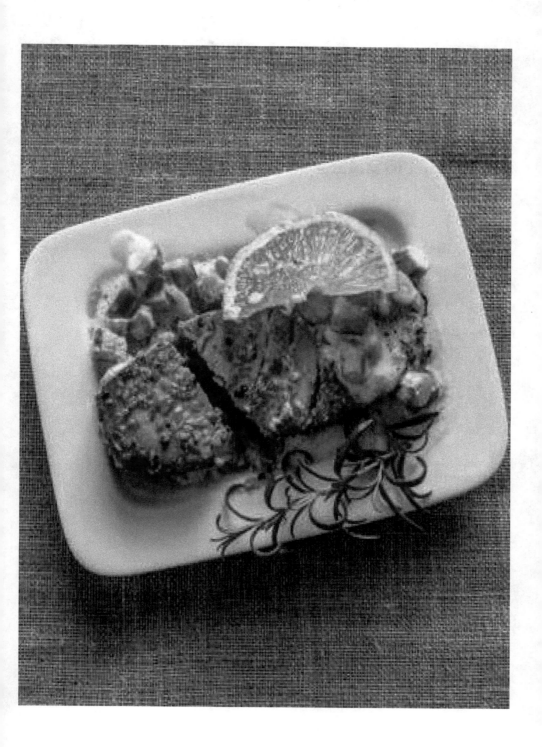

Salmon Egg Salad

Preparation Time: 5 Minutes

Cooking Time: 5 Minutes

Total Time: 10 Minutes

Serves: 2

Ingredients

- 2 hard-boiled eggs -
- ¼ cup red onion -
- 2 tablespoons capers -
- 1 tablespoon lime juice -
- 3 oz. smoked salmon -
- 1 tablespoon olive oil

Instructions

1. In a bowl combine all ingredients together and mix well
2. Serve with dressing

Baked Lemon Salmon

Preparation Time: 10 Minutes

Cooking Time: 20 Minutes

Total Time: 30 Minutes

Serves: 1

Ingredients

- 1 zucchini -
- 1 onion -
- 1 scallion -
- 1 salmon fillet -
- 1 tsp lemon zest -
- 1 tsp olive oil -
- Lemon slices

Instructions

1. Preheat the oven to 375 F
2. In a baking dish add zucchini, onion and sprinkle vegetables with salt and lemon zest
3. Lay salmon fillet and season with salt, lemon zest and olive oil
4. Bake at 375 F for 15-18 minutes
5. When ready remove from the oven and serve with lemon slices

Rutabaga Hash

Preparation Time: 10 Minutes

Cooking Time: 20 Minutes

Total Time: 30 Minutes

Serves: 2

Ingredients

- 2 tablespoons olive oil -
- 1 rutabaga -
- ¼ cup onion -
- ¼ cup red pepper -
- 1 tsp salt -
- ¼ tsp black pepper

Instructions

1. In a skillet heat olive oil and fry rutabaga for 3-4 minutes
2. Cook for another 5-6 minutes or until rutabaga is tender
3. Add onion, red pepper, black pepper, salt and stir to combine
4. Garnish with dill and serve

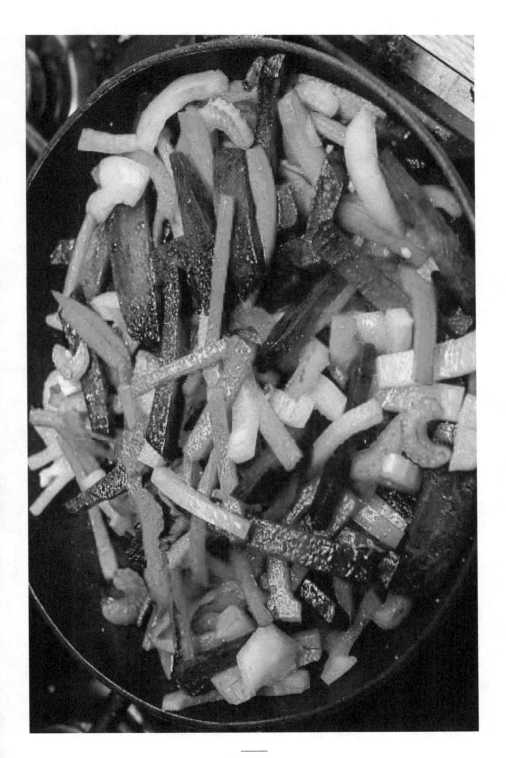

CPSIA information can be obtained
at www.ICGtesting.com
Printed in the USA
LVHW051034230621
690925LV00005B/392